CIALIS

"(strong Tada-la-fil)"

A Guide To Conquer Erectile Dysfunction
And Revitalize Your Intimacy, Passion,
Confidence And Reignite Your Desires while
Enhancing Your Sexual Performance

Dr. Gerald Paul

1

Table of Contents

Section 1 3

UNDERSTANDING THE FUNDAMENTALS OF

CIALIS: CIALIS: WHAT IS IT? 3

What is Cialis's Effect?......................................5

Section 2 9

THE ADVANTAGES OF CIALIS...........................9

Enhancing Well-Being: Mental and Close to

home Advantages...12

Section 3 16

CIALIS MEASUREMENTS AND ORGANIZATION

....16

Administration orally: Instructions to Take

Cialis 18

Factors Influencing Cialis Retention and

Adequacy...19

Section 4..23

SECURITY AND PRECAUTIONARY MEASURES 23

Section 5..31

LIFESTYLE FACTORS THAT INCREASE CIALIS'

EFFECTIVENESS...............................31

Planning And Timing: When To Take Cialis To

Get The Most Out Of Cialis...........................33

Section 6..38

COMMON MISPERCEPTIONS AND QUESTIONS

ABOUT CIALIS 38

Will Cialis Make Me Want To Have Sex More?

....38

Could I At Any Point Take Cialis Assuming I

Have Fundamental Ailments? 39

Concerns About Cialis's Safety and

Effectiveness Is it safe to use?......................40

Authentic Discussions: 42

What issues should I bring up with my doctor?

....42

Section 7 45

ELECTIVE MEDICINES FOR ERECTILE

BROKENNESS...45

Section 8 50

A COMPREHENSIVE WAY TO DEAL WITH

SEXUAL HEALTH...50

Intimacy and Interaction: Fortifying

Connections...53

Conclusion 57

EMBRACING THE FORCE OF CIALIS FOR A

SATISFYING LIFE 57

Section 1

UNDERSTANDING THE FUNDAMENTALS OF CIALIS: CIALIS: WHAT IS IT?

Both erectile dysfunction (ED) and benign prostatic hyperplasia (BPH), also known as an enlarged prostate gland, can be treated with the medication Cialis. It has a place with a class of medications called phosphodiesterase type 5 (PDE5) inhibitors. The dynamic fixing in Cialis is tadalafil.

Cialis can be purchased as a tablet in a variety of strengths, including 2.5 mg, 5 mg, 10 mg, and 20 mg. The drug is normally taken orally, regardless of food, as coordinated by a medical services proficient.

Cialis' Development and History:

The pharmaceutical company ICOS Corporation and Eli Lilly and Company began developing a drug to treat erectile dysfunction in the late 1990s, which is when Cialis was developed. The goal was to develop a medication with a longer half-life than other ED treatments currently available.

In 2003, the U.S. Food and Drug Administration (FDA) granted Cialis approval as a prescription medication for the treatment of erectile dysfunction (ED). This approval followed years of research and clinical trials. It later got extra endorsements for the treatment of BPH and a blend of ED and BPH.

What is Cialis's Effect?

Cialis works by restraining the chemical phosphodiesterase type 5 (PDE5). Cyclic guanosine monophosphate (cGMP), a chemical that encourages relaxation of smooth muscles and increased blood flow to the penis, is broken down by PDE5.

At the point when a man is physically animated, the arrival of nitric oxide (NO) in the penis causes an expansion in cGMP levels. This causes the smooth muscles in the penile arteries to relax, allowing more blood to flow into the erectile tissues, which in turn causes an erection.

Cialis helps to maintain higher levels of cGMP in the penis by inhibiting PDE5, which extends the duration of the erection. It doesn't straightforwardly cause an erection yet upgrades the regular course of sexual excitement.

It's important to remember that Cialis does not make you want or feel more sexual. In order for the medication to be effective, sexual stimulation is still required.

Cialis has a more drawn out length of activity contrasted with other PDE5 inhibitors, like sildenafil (Viagra) and vardenafil (Levitra). The fact that it can improve erectile function for up to 36 hours has earned it the moniker "the weekend pill." Because the medication does not need to be taken immediately prior to sexual activity, this extended window of effectiveness allows for greater spontaneity in sexual activity.

Cialis is approved for the treatment of BPH in addition to its use to treat erectile dysfunction (ED). In this instance, the medication reduces symptoms of an enlarged prostate gland and improves urinary flow by relaxing the smooth muscles in the bladder and prostate.

Cialis should be taken as directed by a healthcare professional, and the dosage and usage instructions should be followed. Cialis should not be taken more frequently than once per day.

Although not everyone experiences side effects, Cialis may cause them, as with any medication. Normal incidental effects might incorporate migraine, heartburn, muscle hurts, back torment, and nasal blockage. Serious secondary effects are interesting however may incorporate priapism (a drawn out and difficult erection enduring over four hours) or unexpected vision misfortune.

It is critical to talk with a medical care proficient prior to beginning Cialis or some other prescription, as they can give customized direction in light of individual ailments and drugs being taken.

Section 2

THE ADVANTAGES OF CIALIS

Upgrading Erectile Capability: Erectile Dysfunction Treatment The effectiveness of Cialis in treating erectile dysfunction (ED) is one of its primary advantages. Erectile brokenness is a typical condition portrayed by the failure to accomplish or keep an erection adequate for palatable sexual execution. By increasing blood flow to the penis, Cialis helps improve erectile function, resulting in a firm and long-lasting erection.

Among Cialis' benefits for treating ED are:

Enhancement of Sexual Performance: Cialis can fundamentally improve sexual execution by aiding men accomplish and keep up with erections. This can prompt expanded certainty, fulfillment, and closeness in sexual connections.

Increased Flexibility: Cialis has a longer half-life than some other ED medications, which must be taken shortly before sexual activity. As a result, men are able to take Cialis ahead of time and have a wider window of opportunity for sexual activity, resulting in more spontaneity and less pressure to have sexual encounters at specific times.

Enhanced Partners' Sexual Satisfaction: Additionally, men with ED's partners may benefit from Cialis. By empowering a more dependable and longer-enduring erection, Cialis can work on the by and large sexual experience for the two accomplices, prompting expanded fulfillment and closeness in the relationship.

Past ED: Cialis's Other Medical Applications In addition to being used to treat erectile dysfunction, Cialis can also be used to treat pulmonary arterial hypertension (PAH) and benign prostatic hyperplasia (BPH).

BPH, or benign prostatic hyperplasia, is Cialis is endorsed for the therapy of BPH, which is a non-malignant extension of the prostate organ. Cialis improves urinary flow and reduces BPH symptoms like frequent urination, urgency, and weak urine stream by relaxing the smooth muscles in the bladder and prostate.

Pneumonic Blood vessel Hypertension (PAH): Additionally, Cialis is used to treat PAH, which is characterized by elevated blood pressure in the arteries that supply the lungs. By loosening up the smooth muscles in the aspiratory veins, Cialis further develops blood stream and decreases the responsibility on the heart, prompting further developed practice limit and personal satisfaction for people with PAH.

Enhancing Well-Being: Mental and Close to home Advantages

Past its actual impacts, Cialis can likewise have mental and close to home advantages for people with ED or different circumstances. These advantages can essentially affect a singular's general personal satisfaction and prosperity:

Expanded Certainty: Cialis can help fearlessness and confidence in men with ED by furnishing them with the affirmation that they can accomplish and keep an erection when required. Having a more relaxed and enjoyable sexual experience is made possible by this, which can reduce anxiety and stress related to performance.

Worked on Profound Prosperity: A person's mental and emotional health can be negatively impacted by erectile dysfunction, which can cause feelings of anger, shame, and even depression. By successfully treating ED, Cialis can assist with lightening these gloomy feelings and add to worked on close to home prosperity and a more inspirational perspective on life.

Enhanced Relationships and Intimacy: An important factor in intimacy and overall relationship satisfaction is a sexual relationship that is satisfying. By working on erectile capability and sexual execution, Cialis can fortify the close to home connection among accomplices and upgrade closeness, prompting a seriously satisfying and charming relationship.

It is essential to keep in mind that, despite its numerous benefits, Cialis is not a treatment for erectile dysfunction or any other medical condition. To address any underlying health issues and determine the appropriate use of Cialis, it is essential to consult a medical professional.

Furthermore, likely secondary effects and connections with different drugs ought to be examined with a medical services supplier to guarantee protected and successful utilization of Cialis

Section 3

CIALIS MEASUREMENTS AND ORGANIZATION

Tracking down the Right Measurements: Figuring out the Choices

Cialis is accessible in various measurements, and finding the right dose is significant for ideal adequacy and wellbeing. The individual's medical condition, response to treatment, and any other medications they may be taking all play a role in determining the appropriate dosage. For the best Cialis dosage, you should talk to a doctor or other medical professional.

Doses for Cialis are as follows:

2.5 mg and 5 mg: Typically, these lower doses are taken every day. They are good for people who have more than two sexual encounters per week and would rather not have to take a medication every day.

10 mg and 20 mg: Typically, these higher doses are used as needed. They are taken before expected sexual action, ordinarily around 30 minutes to 1 hour prior. Although the higher dose may be more effective for some people, it also carries a higher risk of side effects.

When determining the appropriate dosage, the healthcare professional will take into account the severity of the condition, individual health, and response to the medication.

Administration orally: Instructions to Take Cialis

Cialis is typically taken orally, regardless of food, as coordinated by a medical services proficient. It is absolutely necessary to carefully observe the dosage and administration instructions. The tablets should not be broken, chewed, or crushed; they should be swallowed whole with a glass of water.

For day to day use measurements (2.5 mg and 5 mg), Cialis can be taken at roughly a similar time consistently, paying little heed to sexual action. The body will always have the same amount of the medication because of this.

Cialis should be taken before anticipated sexual activity in the as-needed dosages of 10 mg and 20 mg, respectively. It is essential to keep in mind that sexual activity is still required for the medication to be effective. Taking Cialis 30 minutes to 1 hour before engaging in sexual activity is generally recommended, though the exact timing of administration may vary depending on individual response.

Factors Influencing Cialis Retention and Adequacy

A few elements can impact the ingestion and viability of Cialis. People can get the most out of their medication if they are aware of these factors:

Food Admission: Taking Cialis with a dinner, particularly a high-fat feast, may defer the beginning of activity. Consuming foods high in fat may hinder the medication's absorption, reducing its effectiveness. For best results, Cialis is typically taken on an empty stomach or with a light meal.

Beverage consumption: Savoring liquor abundance can disable sexual capability and diminish the adequacy of Cialis. When taking Cialis, it is best to drink only a small amount or not at all.

Conditions and Prescription Drugs: Cialis can be adversely affected or interact with other medications and medical conditions. To ensure that Cialis is used safely and effectively, it is essential to tell your doctor about all of your current medications, including herbal supplements and those purchased over the counter. People with basic ailments, like cardiovascular infection, liver or kidney debilitation, or retinitis pigmentosa, ought to likewise uncover their clinical history to the medical services proficient.

Metabolism and age: More seasoned people might require lower dosages of Cialis because of expected age-related changes in drug digestion and freedom. The medical care proficient will consider these variables while deciding the fitting dose.

It is essential to keep in mind that no matter the dosage, Cialis should only be taken once per day. Taking beyond what the recommended portion can expand the gamble of aftereffects without giving extra advantages.

In the event that any troubles or concerns emerge while taking Cialis, it is vital to talk with a medical services proficient for direction. They can give customized guidance and change the measurements if important to guarantee the best result.

Section 4

SECURITY AND PRECAUTIONARY MEASURES

Normal Symptoms of Cialis

While Cialis is by and large very much endured, similar to any drug, it can cause secondary effects. Not every person encounters aftereffects, and the seriousness and event of secondary effects might shift among people. Common Cialis side effects include:

Headache: People who take Cialis frequently report experiencing headaches as a side effect. These headaches typically range in severity from mild to moderate and may improve over time as the body gets used to the medication.

Acid reflux and Agitated Stomach: After taking Cialis, some people may experience indigestion, acid reflux, or stomach pain. This can appear as stomach uneasiness, swelling, or acid reflux.

Back and muscle pain: Muscle hurts and back torment are expected symptoms of Cialis. These side effects are commonly gentle and transient, settling all alone without clinical mediation.

Flushing and Nasal Clog: Facial flushing, characterized by warmth and redness in the face and neck, can be caused by Cialis. A stuffy or congested nose is another possibility.

Changes in Vision: In uncommon cases, people might encounter impermanent changes in vision, including obscured vision, changes in variety discernment, or expanded aversion to light. It is essential to seek medical attention right away if any vision changes occur.

It's important to remember that these side effects are typically mild and short-lived. However, it is best to seek further evaluation from a healthcare professional if any side effects persist or become bothersome.

Identifying Potential Drug Interactions Cialis can interact with some drugs, which can make it less effective or make it more likely to cause side effects. It is essential to inform the physician of all medications being taken, including herbal supplements and prescription and over-the-counter medications. Cialis may interact with the following medications:

Nitrates: It is not recommended to take Cialis at the same time as nitrates or nitric oxide donors (like nitroglycerin), as this can result in a significant drop in blood pressure and potentially serious side effects.

Alpha-Blockers: Watchfulness ought to be practiced while joining Cialis with alpha-blockers, as the two prescriptions can bring down pulse. To reduce the likelihood of symptomatic hypotension, a dose adjustment may be required.

Other PDE5 Inhibitors: Avoid using multiple PDE5 inhibitors at the same time, such as sildenafil (Viagra) and vardenafil (Levitra), as this can increase the likelihood of side effects.

CYP3A4 Inhibitors: The body's concentration of Cialis can be increased by taking certain medications that inhibit the enzyme CYP3A4, such as ketoconazole and itraconazole, which are antifungal medications, and ritonavir and saquinavir, which are HIV protease inhibitors.

During Cialis treatment, it is essential to follow the healthcare provider's instructions regarding potential drug interactions and to notify them of any medication changes.

Special Considerations for Patients with Pre-Existing Conditions When taking Cialis, patients with particular pre-existing conditions should exercise caution. To ensure the medication is used safely and appropriately, it is essential to disclose any underlying health conditions to the healthcare provider. Among the special considerations are:

Disease of the Heart: Due to the potential risk of cardiovascular complications associated with sexual activity, individuals who have a history of cardiovascular disease, such as heart disease, stroke, or angina, should use Cialis with caution. The medical services proficient will assess the person's cardiovascular wellbeing and decide whether Cialis is appropriate.

Liver or Kidney Weakness: Cialis ought to be involved with alert in people with liver or kidney hindrance. Portion changes might be vital in light of the seriousness of the disability.

Pigmentary retinitis: Cialis should be used with caution by people who have the rare genetic eye disorder retinitis pigmentosa because there have been very few reports of this condition causing vision loss.

Priapism: Priapism, a delayed and difficult erection enduring over four hours, is an interesting however possibly serious symptom of Cialis. People with a background marked by priapism or conditions inclining them toward priapism, like sickle cell sickliness or leukemia, ought to utilize Cialis with mindfulness and look for guaranteed clinical consideration on the off chance that an erection endures longer than four hours.

Allergies: People with known sensitivities or extreme touchiness to tadalafil or some other parts of Cialis ought to keep away from its utilization.

Before beginning Cialis, it is essential to fully discuss any pre-existing conditions or concerns with a medical professional. The medical services proficient can give customized exhortation and direction in light of individual conditions to guarantee protected and successful utilization of the drug.

Section 5

LIFESTYLE FACTORS THAT INCREASE CIALIS' EFFECTIVENESS

Solid Propensities for Further developed Results

While Cialis can be powerful in treating erectile brokenness (ED), consolidating solid way of life propensities can additionally upgrade its adequacy. When taking Cialis, the following lifestyle factors may help you get better results:

Regular sport: Participating in standard actual work has been displayed to work on erectile capability. Sexual health can benefit from exercise because it improves cardiovascular health, reduces stress, and promotes healthy blood circulation. At least 150 minutes a week of moderate-intensity aerobic exercise, such as cycling, brisk walking, or jogging, should be your goal.

Healthy Diet: A healthy, well-balanced diet is important for everything, including sexual health. Consolidate different organic products, vegetables, entire grains, lean proteins, and sound fats into your eating routine. Consuming a lot of alcohol, sugary snacks, and processed foods can have a negative impact on sexual function.

Controlling your weight: For optimal sexual function, it is important to keep a healthy weight. Heftiness is related with expanded chance of ED and other ailments that can add to sexual challenges. A healthy weight should be your goal through regular exercise and a well-balanced diet.

Stress Management: Ongoing pressure can slow down sexual capability. Practice pressure the board procedures, like contemplation, profound breathing activities, yoga, or taking part in side interests and exercises that you appreciate. Getting help from a therapist or counselor can also help you manage stress and feel better all around.

Planning And Timing: When To Take Cialis To Get The Most Out Of Cialis.

Adhere to Medical services Proficient's Guidelines: Continuously stick to the recommended measurement and timing guidelines given by your medical services proficient. When determining when to take Cialis, they will take into account your medical condition, response to treatment, and any other medications you may be taking.

Prepare: Plan your sexual activities in advance if you are taking Cialis in as-needed doses. Take the prescription around 30 minutes to 1 hour before expected sexual action to permit adequate time for the drug to produce results. This can help make sure that you and your partner can have sex when you want to.

Stay away from High-Fat Dinners: Consuming Cialis with a meal high in fat may delay its effects. Cialis should be taken on an empty stomach or with a light meal to be of maximum benefit. Diets high in fat have the potential to hinder the medication's absorption and effectiveness.

Joining Cialis with Different Medicines: A Comprehensive Approach Sometimes, Cialis can be more effective when combined with other treatments or interventions to provide a comprehensive approach to erectile dysfunction. Think about the following choices:

Psychological Therapy: Erectile brokenness can have mental causes or add to profound misery. Participating in advising or treatment, either exclusively or with your accomplice, can assist with tending to hidden mental factors and work on sexual capability.

Different Meds: In specific cases, consolidating Cialis with different drugs might be helpful. For instance, managing and treating an underlying health condition, such as diabetes or high blood pressure, in conjunction with Cialis can improve overall sexual health.

Penile Implants or Vacuum Equipment: Vacuum erection devices or penile implants may be considered if oral medications are ineffective or inconvenient. These gadgets can help accomplish and keep an erection, giving another option or extra treatment choice for people with ED.

It's important to talk to a doctor or other medical professional about whether or not Cialis should be used in conjunction with other treatments and how to proceed based on your specific circumstances.

In synopsis, expanding the viability of Cialis includes taking on sound way of life propensities, including standard activity, a decent eating routine, stress decrease methods, and keeping a solid weight. Cialis can also be more effective if you take it as directed, plan your sexual activities ahead of time, and follow the dosage and timing instructions. Erectile dysfunction treatment may be more comprehensive when Cialis is used in conjunction with other medications or treatments, such as psychological counseling. It is critical to work intimately with a medical services proficient to guarantee protected and viable utilization of Cialis and to fit the therapy plan to individual necessities.

Section 6

COMMON MISPERCEPTIONS AND QUESTIONS ABOUT CIALIS

Is Cialis a Solution to Erectile Dysfunction (ED)?

Cialis does not provide ED relief. By increasing blood flow to the penis, it is a medication that aids in improving erectile function. It temporarily alleviates ED symptoms without addressing the underlying causes. If you want to find the best course of treatment for your particular situation, it's important to talk to a medical professional.

Will Cialis Make Me Want To Have Sex More?

No, Cialis does not make you want to get sexual. When sexually stimulated, it helps you achieve and maintain an erection and improves erectile function. Personal factors and experiences continue to influence sexual desire and arousal.

Could I At Any Point Take Cialis Assuming I Have Fundamental Ailments?

Cialis can be utilized by people with specific fundamental ailments, however it is critical to talk with a medical care proficient prior to beginning the prescription. They will look at your medical history and figure out if Cialis is safe for you and what you should do. To ensure safe use, it is essential to disclose all medical conditions and medications.

Concerns About Cialis's Safety and Effectiveness Is it safe to use?

Cialis is generally regarded as safe when taken according to directions and under medical supervision. However, not everyone might find it useful. To ensure that your medications and underlying medical conditions are safe and effective for you, it is essential to inform your healthcare provider. They will take into account your particular circumstances and weigh the potential benefits and risks.

How long does Cialis take to work?

The time it takes for Cialis to start working varies from person to person and from dose to dose. For most people, Cialis begins working in something like 30 minutes to 1 hour after organization. However, sexual activity is still necessary for the medication to work.

Is Cialis safe and effective for men who have erectile dysfunction?

Numerous men with erectile dysfunction have seen success with Cialis. Be that as it may, individual reactions might fluctuate. Factors like the fundamental reason for ED, generally speaking wellbeing, and individual contrasts can impact the viability of Cialis. It is critical to work intimately with a medical care proficient to decide the most suitable therapy approach for your particular circumstance.

Authentic Discussions:
Having a Conversation with Your Doctor Why Should I Talk to My Doctor About Cialis?

If you want to use Cialis safely and effectively, it's important to talk to your doctor about it. They can survey your clinical history, assess likely dangers and advantages, and decide the fitting measurement and treatment plan for your particular necessities. They can likewise address any worries or questions you might have and give customized direction.

What issues should I bring up with my doctor?

It is essential to discuss your medical history with your healthcare provider, including any underlying health conditions, medications, or allergies. Illuminate them about your side effects regarding erectile brokenness and any past medicines you might have attempted. Be transparent about your interests, assumptions, and sexual wellbeing objectives. This will assist your medical services supplier with pursuing informed choices and give the most ideal consideration.

Might I at any point raise touchy themes with my medical care supplier?

Absolutely. It is critical to have open and authentic discussions with your medical services supplier, particularly while talking about delicate subjects like sexual wellbeing. They are experts prepared to address these themes in a conscious and non-critical way. You make it possible for them to provide the appropriate care and direction that is tailored to your requirements by providing information that is truthful and accurate.

Keep in mind that your doctor or nurse is the best person to talk to about Cialis and your overall health and is there to assist you.

Open correspondence can prompt a superior comprehension of your particular circumstance and guarantee that you get the most reasonable consideration.

Section 7

ELECTIVE MEDICINES FOR ERECTILE BROKENNESS

Investigating Non-Remedy Choices

Vacuum Erection Gadgets: Non-prescription vacuum erection devices (VEDs) draw blood into the erectile tissues and induce an erection by creating a vacuum around the penis. A cylinder that is positioned over the penis and a pump that removes air from the cylinder make up these devices. When an erection is accomplished, a choking ring is set at the foundation of the penis to keep up with the erection.

Penile Inserts: Penile implants are surgical devices inserted into the penis to facilitate erections and their maintenance. Penile implants can be of two main types: inflatable inserts and moldable inserts. A pump is inserted into the scrotum of an inflatable implant, which allows the user to manually inflate or deflate the device. The reservoir is filled with fluid. Rods called malleable implants are inserted into the penis through a surgical procedure, allowing it to be bent into an erect or flaccid position.

Natural treatments and modifications to one's way of life Healthy habits: Erectile function can be improved by leading a healthy lifestyle. This includes doing regular exercise, eating a healthy diet, keeping a healthy weight, managing stress, and avoiding smoking and drinking too much alcohol.

Exercises for the Pelvis: Kegel exercises, also known as exercises for the pelvic floor, can help strengthen the muscles necessary for erectile function. Erectile function can be improved by performing these exercises, which involve contracting and relaxing the pelvic floor muscles.

Medicinal Herbs: L-arginine, ginseng, and horny goat weed, among other herbal supplements, have been suggested as potential treatments for erectile dysfunction. However, these supplements' safety and efficacy are not well-established, so it's important to talk to a doctor before using them.

Other Physician endorsed Drugs for ED

Beside Cialis (tadalafil), there are other physician endorsed drugs accessible for the treatment of erectile brokenness. These include:

Viagra's Sildenafil: Similar to Cialis, Viagra is another popular PDE5 inhibitor. It is taken as needed, between 30 and 60 minutes before sexual activity. A medical professional should direct you to follow the dosage and usage instructions.

Levitra (vardenafil): Additionally, erectile dysfunction can be treated with Levitra, which is a PDE5 inhibitor. It is ordinarily taken dependent upon the situation, roughly 1 hour before sexual movement. Like other PDE5 inhibitors, the measurement and organization ought to be followed as recommended.

Stendra (Avanafil): Avanafil is a more recent PDE5 inhibitor that can be taken as needed. It is by and large taken around 15 to 30 minutes before sexual movement. Follow the dosage and timing instructions as directed by a medical professional.

When trying to treat erectile dysfunction, it's important to talk to a doctor or other medical professional. They are able to evaluate your particular circumstance, take into account things like underlying health conditions and medication interactions, and offer advice on the treatment strategy that will work best for you.

Section 8

A COMPREHENSIVE WAY TO DEAL WITH SEXUAL HEALTH

Past Prescription: Developing a Comprehensive Sexual Health Plan When it comes to promoting sexual health, a comprehensive strategy that goes beyond medication is essential. A variety of physical, emotional, and interpersonal well-being aspects are included in a comprehensive sexual health plan. The following are important considerations:

Normal Check-ups: Normal visits to a medical care proficient are fundamental for keeping up with generally wellbeing and tending to any potential basic ailments that might influence sexual health. This includes reviewing medication and treatment options, having discussions about sexual health issues, and conducting routine screenings.

Solid Way of life Propensities: Sexual health can be positively impacted by leading a healthy lifestyle. This includes exercising on a regular basis, eating a well-balanced diet, controlling stress, getting enough sleep, and avoiding smoking and drinking too much alcohol. These way of life propensities advance by and large prosperity and can improve sexual capability.

Intimacy and Interaction: Transparent correspondence with your accomplice is indispensable for a solid sexual relationship. A feeling of emotional intimacy and connection is created when boundaries, concerns, and desires are expressed. The bond between partners can be strengthened and sexual satisfaction enhanced by talking about sexual expectations, trying new things, and learning about each other's needs.

Mental and Close to home Prosperity: Sexual health is significantly influenced by mental and emotional well-being. Stress, nervousness, misery, and other mental elements can influence sexual capability. Taking part in pressure the board procedures, looking for treatment or guiding when required, and focusing on taking care of oneself can work on mental and close to home prosperity, prompting better sexual encounters.

Resources and instruction: Finding reliable resources and educating yourself about sexual health can provide helpful information and support. There are various trustworthy sources, books, sites, and associations committed to sexual wellbeing that offer direction on a scope of points, including sexual life structures, delight, contraception, and sexual problems.

Intimacy and Interaction: Fortifying Connections

Open and Non-critical Correspondence: When you talk to your partner in an open and non-judgmental way, you create a safe environment where you can talk about your sexual desires, concerns, and boundaries. Undivided attention, sympathy, and communicating appreciation for one another's requirements encourage understanding and association.

Quality Time: Spend quality time with your partner without engaging in sexual activity. Participate in exercises that you both appreciate, like shared side interests, excursions, or even straightforward discussions over a dinner. Building profound closeness and keeping serious areas of strength for an association improves sexual fulfillment.

Experimentation and Research: Be available to investigating new encounters and sexual exercises with your accomplice. This may entail experimenting with novel strategies and positions, introducing toys, or role-playing. When looking into new aspects of intimacy, open communication and mutual consent are essential.

Mental and Close to home Prosperity: Self-care is crucial for stress management: Participate in pressure decreasing exercises like activity, reflection, profound breathing activities, or participating in side interests and exercises that give you pleasure and unwinding. Make time for self-care and activities that support your mental and emotional health.

Getting Help: Seek support from a mental health professional if you are experiencing difficulties or mental health issues that impact your overall well-being. Treatment or directing can give a place of refuge to resolve hidden intense subject matters that might influence sexual wellbeing.

Self-Exploration: Sexual health depends on having a clear understanding of your own needs, preferences, and boundaries. Take part in self-investigation, find out about your body, and embrace self-delight. Self-awareness can boost sexual confidence and make it easier to talk to your partner.

Keep in mind, sexual wellbeing envelops physical, close to home, and social parts of life. A more fulfilling and satisfying sexual life can be achieved by adopting a holistic approach that includes self-care, intimate connection, and open communication. Make it a point to proficient direction and backing when expected to address explicit worries or difficulties you might experience en route.

Conclusion:

EMBRACING THE FORCE OF CIALIS FOR A SATISFYING LIFE

Cialis is a strong prescription that has changed the existences of numerous people encountering erectile brokenness and other related conditions. Through its instrument of activity, Cialis works on erectile capability, permitting people to recapture sexual certainty and improve their general personal satisfaction. Cialis enables individuals to engage in sexual activities on their terms thanks to its longer duration of action and adaptable dosing options.

Nevertheless, it is essential to acknowledge that Cialis is not a stand-alone treatment. It is only one part of a comprehensive strategy for sexual health. Embracing a comprehensive point of view includes tending to way of life factors, participating in open correspondence with accomplices, focusing on mental and profound prosperity, and looking for proficient help when important.

Individuals can further enhance the effectiveness of Cialis and improve overall sexual function by incorporating healthy lifestyle habits like regular exercise, a balanced diet, stress management, and maintaining a healthy weight. Correspondence and closeness assume a crucial part in cultivating fulfilling connections, while focusing on mental and profound prosperity adds to a positive outlook and sexual certainty.

It is urgent to recall that each individual's involvement in Cialis might shift, and it is vital to talk with a medical care proficient to decide the most proper therapy approach in view of individual requirements, medical issue, and objectives. They are able to provide you with individualized direction, monitor your progress, and address any issues or inquiries that may arise.

Individuals can reclaim their sexual vitality, experience greater intimacy and satisfaction in their relationships, and embrace a life that is satisfying and fulfilling with the power of Cialis and a holistic approach to sexual wellness.

Made in United States
Troutdale, OR
02/03/2024

17427916R00037